THE ANXIETY CHECK-IN

A Guided Journal to Support Your Mental Health and Help You Through the Hard Days

BREE CARTWRIGHT

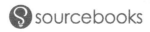

Published by Sourcebooks
P.O. Box 4410, Naperville, Illinois 60567-4410
(630) 961-3900
sourcebooks.com

Printed and bound in the United States of America.
POD 10 9 8 7 6 5 4 3 2 1

INTRODUCTION

So Maybe It Isn't So Fine Right Now (but It Will Be)

So...things are kind of a shit show right now, huh?

Welcome!

To start things off, you should know that managing your mental health is damn hard. The world sucks sometimes, and it's easy to feel like you're all alone, trying to get it together. But you're *not* alone. Everyone has days (or weeks or months) where they don't feel all right. It's not a fun place to be, and it can feel overwhelming. Don't worry! You're doing the right thing by starting this journal, the first of many steps in a more positive, productive direction.

This journal is designed to help you identify the warning signs of a shit storm and gather the tools you need to weather it. If you're in a state where opening your kitchen drawer and finding zero clean forks has you on the verge of tears, it's not about the forks. The better you get at checking in with yourself, the better you'll get at identifying your triggers big and small—and that's how this journal will help. Maybe those dirty forks really are simply the end of your patience. But maybe you're at your wits' end because you are already spending a shit-ton of energy to get out of bed in the morning, to put a smile on, to figure out why you feel so bad...and the forks are just one more unexpected wrench in your plan.

No matter where you are in your journey, there will be bad days. And this journal will be here for you when shit is really hitting the fan. Sometimes, just screaming into the void, or onto the page, is enough. Other times you'll need to call in the heavy hitters from your support network. Either way, the prompts in this book will help you manage the tough times and achieve actual wellness.

Scary as it may seem, you're embarking on a kick-ass journey here. Getting your mental health on track can make all the difference in your life. How much can you accomplish without anxiety whispering in your ear about everything that could go wrong? What opportunities will you be able to take on when you're not trapped thinking about your past mistakes? Not to mention, when you make space for self-care and self-love, you teach yourself and the world that you're worthy and downright deserving of good things. You're expected to spend all kinds of time and energy on getting your body in shape. How about devoting some of that attention to your mental state?

As you work your way through this journal, don't stress about doing things in order. Each section tackles a different aspect of taming your brain gremlins. If you want to start at the first page and work through the prompts as they come, follow that bliss. But if you need some of the later pages right now, skip on ahead. It's *your* mental health, so you get to pick how to unfuck your mind.

Most of all, know that feeling like garbage is not the end. Mental health is an ongoing struggle, but you have the strength to build your resilience, manage your stress, and bring wellness into your life. Go ahead, lose your shit, then come back to this journal to dust yourself off and move forward.

WELLNESS

Welcome to the Shit Show

Mental health is a moving target, so where do you even start? This chapter will take you through some self-assessment and goal setting. You wouldn't be here if you felt great, but how close are you to a total meltdown? Are you just starting to notice that you're clenching your teeth? Have you been one missed cup of coffee away from a screaming fit all week? When did you last take a deep breath?

Once you establish where you are, think about where you *want* to be. "Feeling good" doesn't mean the same thing to everyone, so this is your chance to decide where you want to end up. Do you want to skip across town singing? Do you just want to spend a whole day without hearing phantom sirens in your head? Today's finish line is up to you.

Before you get too far, though, take a second and congratulate yourself. You've already made it here. You know a ton of things that work for you (and all the shit that doesn't). Don't forget that you're already doing the damn thing, and you deserve some acknowledgment. You, and hundreds of other people out there, have decided to take some time out of your hectic life to prioritize your wellness. You should be so proud of yourself.

Let's start off easy. How do you feel today? On a scale of one (complete shit) to ten (pretty damn great), how has your mental health been?

Draw a circle in the center of the page. Then, draw a face that represents your current mental state. In the space outside the circle, list the factors contributing to your mental health. Leave it all out on the page.

What are your wellness goals? What do you want to accomplish in the next week, month, and year?

How do you know when you're about to
lose your shit? What does it feel like?

List ten triggers that negatively affect your mental health. Next to it, list ten things you can do that have a positive influence in your life.

What does self-care mean to you? When was
the last time you engaged in true self-care?

Free write a list of all your favorite self-care techniques. They can be big (taking a long-ass vacation) or small (wearing your favorite socks)—just fill the damn page with all the ways you can foster wellness in your life.

How has your mental health evolved over the years?

How would you like to grow in the next year?

Take stock of your current mental state. What do you
need right now? How are you physically feeling?

Make a list of ten things you've achieved despite your struggles with your mental health. Now, list ten things you still want to achieve. How can you get there?

What subtle (or not so subtle) signs do you see

when you're starting to really struggle?

Make a list of all your coping mechanisms. Rank them from one (works, I guess?) to ten (my lifeline).

What unhealthy coping mechanism have you used? What's a healthier alternative?

Do you feel like you have a solid support system?

If not, how can you start building one today?

What frightens you most about your mental health?

What positive lessons has your journey taught you?

How can you invest in yourself today?

Draw an outline of your brain. Fill it with all the thoughts you've been struggling with lately. What is one thing you can address today?

ANXIETY

Doubts, Fears, and Other Shit You Don't Need

The alarm clock has gone off, and the litany has already started in your head. You've been obsessively clock-watching because you can't be late again. Your chest feels tight, and the air around you seems to have less oxygen than usual. You're worried about your commute, about your friends, about your boss. Everything is going to shit today—you can just feel it. Hello, anxiety!

The problem with anxiety isn't just how shitty it feels when you're stuck in a spiral. It's how easy it is for the fear to start ruling your life and ruining your chances before you even take them. Anxiety can have all kinds of sources, from fear of disappointing your loved ones to your piling to-do list. But it doesn't have to rule you. As you move through these questions, think about how you can stand your ground, even when it means reaching out for something (or someone) to hold on to.

Everyone struggles with fear and doubt. That means everyone is a potential ally as you deal with yours. You don't have to fight your anxiety alone, and the people around you might have some surprising suggestions to keep it from getting the upper hand.

Think about how anxiety feels to you. Draw
a picture that represents your anxiety.

How does anxiety manifest in your body?

Where do you physically feel that tension?

What do you feel most anxious about in this moment?

What is the best-case scenario? Worst-case scenario?

Finally, what is the most realistic scenario?

What are the things that trigger your anxiety?

List ten things that make you anxious. Rate them on a scale of one (that's uncomfortable) to ten (my anxiety is through the roof).

What is one problem you have right now?

What do you need in order to solve it?

How has your anxiety held you back
from living your most fruitful life?

List ten good things that have happened to you this week.

Is there a person or situation currently creating anxiety in your life? Write a letter to that situation to address the conflict.

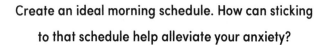

Create an ideal morning schedule. How can sticking
to that schedule help alleviate your anxiety?

Now create your ideal evening routine. Stick to it for five days. Do you notice a difference in your mental state?

List three of your worries across the page. Think about how much influence you have over each one. If there is an actionable course you can take to fix each worry, write the action below. If not, cross it out and put these worries to rest.

What is something that seems out of your control? How does that make you feel?

What would you do if you knew you could

not fail? Write a "bucket list" of ideas.

What is something you need to start saying yes to
and why? What fears are holding you back?

List the questions that are constantly running
through your head. Fill the damn page.
Can you answer just one today?

Visualize a life where you're free from anxiety.

What does that look like? Write the details below.

What support do you need today? Write
down an affirmation to pull you through
the shit storm. Repeat it on the page.

What has living with anxiety taught you? Make a note of three lessons you've learned, either about yourself or others, while coping with your anxiety.

DEPRESSION

Decloud Your Sunshine

Some days there's just a big-ass cloud over your mood, no matter what the weather's like outside. Everyone has days where it seems like too much work to get out of bed. Depression can make it almost impossible to accomplish things, all while telling you that you're not worthwhile if you're not getting anything done. Depression is a damn liar.

No matter how chill and happy the people around you seem, you're not the only one fighting off a depressive funk. Sometimes one small victory, like brushing your teeth, can get the ball rolling. Other times, you may need to take a genuine time-out to recalibrate your misfiring brain. Everyone has a different reset level, but you can build a list of strategies that help no matter what level of shit you're dealing with.

Pay attention to things that feel like sun through the clouds and try getting rid of things that weigh you down. Know that you *can* feel safe and loved and keep track of when that feels most true. You don't need to see rainbows to feel better, and better is one step closer to feeling good.

How does your body feel when you're depressed? Fill the page with the words you'd use to describe your depression.

What does your depression look like? Describe
the shape, color, size, smell, etc. How does
it act, and what does it say to you?

Think about the last time you felt this way. What
did you do to improve your mental health?

Make a schedule of your ideal day. What activities would you include? Can you do any of them today?

What is something you need to let go of?

Why are you holding on to it?

List three things that trigger your depression.

How can you carve them out of your life?

Now, make a list of twenty things, big or small, that bring you joy.

What are three habits that can help improve your mental health? Add them to your calendar for the week. How difficult was it to bring them into your routine? How did you feel after?

What area of your life are you most unhappy with? What are three steps you can take to start improving that area?

How would your life look if you were not depressed?

What differences do you think there would be?

Write ten self-care actions you can take
when you're feeling depressed.

How would you describe depression to someone
who has never experienced it before?

Draw a picture that represents your
perfect life. Is that goal attainable?

List the things you're grateful for in your life. Fill the page with gratitude.

What are some of the triggers of your depression?

How can you avoid those influences?

How do you feel today? Make a list of all the
things you're feeling in this moment. Now,
make a list of how you want to feel.

Who can you talk to when your depression becomes

overwhelming? List three resources to turn to.

Where do you feel safe and loved?

Draw a picture of that space.

What do you wish others knew about

you and your depression?

SELF-AWARENESS
Know Your Damn Self

When you're used to fighting your emotions all day, every day, it's easy to wish they'd simply go away. Not all emotions are bad, though. They can be powerful motivators and guide you to a life you actually love. The more you know about yourself, the more you can use your emotions as a barometer for the decisions you're making. It's about checking in and getting used to feeling all the feelings.

For a lot of people, it's easier to resist having feelings at all than to figure out what to do with them. It's so damn hard to think of a productive use for anger or frustration that a lot of people, maybe even you, avoid any situation that might trigger those feelings. That blocks you off from many rewarding challenges and experiences. So, in order to get the most out of your life, you have to get comfortable with your feels—the good and the bad.

When you know more about your emotions, you can engage with them without feeling like you're about to explode. Buckle up and get ready to be really honest. It's time to break through your discomfort and learn some important shit about yourself.

How do your emotions motivate you? How do they interfere with what you want or need to accomplish?

What are some of the strong emotions you've experienced recently? List them across the page and add an arrow pointing up for a positive emotion or an arrow pointing down for a negative emotion. What does your roller coaster look like?

How do other people impact your emotions?

How do you tend to manage your emotions?

How do you react to your emotions?

Do you find it difficult to talk about
your emotional landscape?

Are you typically aware of how people around you are feeling?

How do you handle conflict? On a scale of one
(please don't yell at me) to ten (I will burn this bridge
to the ground), how confrontational are you?

How would you describe yourself to a stranger?

How does it feel when others succeed around
you? What emotions do you recognize?

What limiting thought recurs in your mind?
How is it holding you back? What would your
life look like if that thought wasn't there?

Think about a time when someone hurt you. If you could say anything to that person, what would you say? Let it out on the page.

On a scale of one (where can I trade this thing in?) to ten (oh damn, I love being me), how happy are you with your life right now? What is influencing that rating?

What does a perfect life look like? List all the things that would make life "perfect."

Let's set some goals. What do you want to accomplish
this year? Where do you want to be in five years? Ten?

List your top five values. How do
those values shape your life?

Think about the last time you felt truly, blissfully happy. Free write about that moment. Where were you? What were you doing? Who were you with?

What kind of world do you want to live in? Make a list of ten "laws" you'd like to enforce in this world. How can you contribute to these ideals?

What is an area of your life you need to work on?

What steps can you take to improve this area?

Draw a picture of yourself. Then fill the page with the values and emotions that define you.

STRESS
Life's Ass-Kicking

All this shit about recognizing your feelings and managing depression and anxiety is well and good. But what do you do when things outside of your control start to go belly-up? You don't necessarily get to decide your work deadlines or when your best friend has a crisis. However, there are still ways you can manage your day-to-day life to make these shit storm moments less panic-inducing.

A big part of managing stress can actually come down to mindfulness. Centering yourself in the present moment can mean a variety of things: acknowledging the thoughts and feelings flying under the surface of your stress, taking a breath to congratulate yourself on a job well done before moving on to the next task, reflecting on your day before bed to calm your worry before you try to sleep. These practices can also help you identify which types of stress are productive and which aren't worth your damn time.

If you're feeling particularly on edge, though, chances are you don't want to do any of that shit. Keep an eye out for warning signs. Was there a noticeable tipping point when your stress became unmanageable? Tweaks to your routine and taking regular time-outs can be a big help in keeping your stress below disaster level.

How do you deal with stress in your life?

How does it tend to manifest?

Free write about a stressful situation you're dealing with. Rant, complain, and vent all over the damn page.

On a scale of one (Zen AF) to ten (stressed to the max), what is your current stress level? What factors are contributing to this rating?

What situations or people feel most stressful to you? What aspects of these situations or people do you have the power to change?

Where do you feel stress in your body? Draw a picture and label all the places you feel stress.

What do you think your stress might be trying to tell you? What area of your life should you reevaluate?

What coping skills do you turn to in times of great stress?

Protecting your time is important during times of stress.
Draw a picture of yourself in the middle of the page.
Then, draw boundaries around yourself and free write
all the things and people you can say no to this week.

Who can you turn to for help when you feel yourself losing your shit? Write their name and number below.

Get organized. Write a to-do list for the day or week and cross off the tasks as you go. How does that structure feel?

Take a time-out and engage in some needed
self-care today. Free journal about the experience.
How did it help with your stress level?

What does perfection mean to you? Do you
expect perfection out of yourself?

Make a list of ten things you excelled at this week.

How can you celebrate these accomplishments?

What are some of your favorite stress-relieving

activities? How do they make you feel?

Dig past your stress for a moment. What are some of the underlying emotions you can recognize? How are those emotions influencing your stress level?

Describe your daily routine. How can you optimize your routine to reduce your stress?

When do you know your stress is
becoming unmanageable? What do you
do when that situation arises?

List some of the negative thoughts you've had
lately. What is at the root of that negativity?

SELF-LOVE

You've Got This!

Here comes the best part...and sometimes the hardest. Time to pony up and love your damn self. No matter how awful things get, you are incredible, and you can conquer your problems. There is so much about you that is worthy of love and happiness, even if it takes some practice to tune in. Keep track of the things that bring you joy, and let those guide your life. Melt your stress with reminders that you are incredible and treat yourself to some positivity—you deserve it.

Before you say it—you're right, it's not that easy. It's common to have to fight down your inner critic before you can give yourself positive attention. You might struggle to find things to be proud of. Acknowledging your flaws is not the end of the road. The end of the road doesn't come until you see that you are both flawed *and* astonishing.

It might help to start small. Hone your sense of joy by thinking about external experiences that make you really happy. Keep looking for that same feeling as you reflect on yourself. With practice, you can start believing the truth: you are radiant.

Draw a heart on the page. Fill it with all the things you love about yourself. Don't leave any white space on the sheet.

List three things you constantly hear from your inner critic. Now draw a line through each and silence that critic for good.

What are five of your best personality traits? What
are five physical features you love about yourself?

What's the weird, random fact you love about yourself?

What do you wish others would know or notice about you?

Let's showcase some self-compassion today. What's one thing you can forgive yourself for? Leave it in the past.

Make a list of ten people whose lives you've positively impacted. Now make a list of ten people who have had a positive impact on your life.

Why do you think you deserve happiness?

How can you fight for your happiest life?

List all of your talents on the page. Now take stock of everything you have to be proud of. Describe how that feels.

Make three columns on the page. In the columns, list the books, movies, and music that make you feel really damn good. Keep them close for a go-to pick-me-up.

What's the best compliment you've ever received, and how did it make you feel?

Name five accomplishments in your life and why
you're proud of yourself for achieving them.

Is there someone you repeatedly compare yourself to? What about that person makes you feel like you can't measure up?

Make a list of ten mistakes you've made in your life. Take a look and finally forgive yourself for these mistakes.

What makes you feel powerful? Fill the page with all the things that fuel your power.

What is your love language? How can you communicate your love language to those around you to feel understood?

What are ten things you're passionate about?

Fill this page with positive affirmations. Every day, recite one that helps you remember that you are enough.

How can you continue to foster joy and wellness in your life? Where do you go from here?

CONCLUSION

You Did the Damn Thing

Your mental health is an ongoing journey. Sometimes you'll feel fine. Sometimes you'll feel terrible but will pretend you feel fine. And sometimes you'll feel better than ever. All of that is normal, and you should celebrate the strides you've taken to take control of your mental health goals. No matter where you land on the spectrum or what you're dealing with today, your mental health is going to be your constant companion. Your anchor to your best, most badass self.

So, guess what?

It's fine.

You're fine.

Actually, you're doing really, really great.